Winning the War on Ticks

LEARN PROVEN COMBAT METHODS FOR PREVENTING TICK BITES

Brian H. Anderson

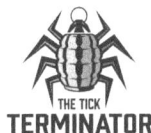

THE TICK
TERMINATOR

The Tick Terminator

Publisher: Brian Anderson

Cover Design by Stacy Hooker

ISBN: 979-8-218-21267-4 (Paperback)

First Edition, 2023

This book is dedicated to my wife Vickie, my family, my friends, and all the business contacts that I meet across the country. It is a joy sharing all the things I have learned about ticks over the last decade of research.

Lyme and other tick-borne diseases are here to stay, so my work on prevention and awareness will never be done!

Contents

Introduction

People always ask me, how did you ever come up with the idea to become The Tick Terminator? I tell them, "Well, you have to be a little weird, a little crazy, and have an unusual fascination with the little blood sucking varmints we call ticks."

It started when I was a kid noticing the little creatures as they sat patiently on a blade of grass waiting to hitch a ride on something and then look for a meal. My wife has always been petrified of them and that fear eventually led to my curiosity to learn even more about them. Around 2010, I finally began with some actual hands-on research that started in my basement. I would bring ticks into the house and play with them on a white carpet just to learn more about what makes them tick. Sometimes I would have my grandkids help me so they could have some fun too. However, one of the big turning points came when a good friend of mine almost died from his struggle with

Lyme disease. This led to not only doing more research in the basement, but a lot more online.

I then realized how much important and helpful information was there for people suffering from Lyme disease but not much about prevention. I guess that is about when I had my "aha" moment. I started thinking how could we keep these darn ticks off from us so we don't get bit in the first place.

This led to the discovery of some great repellants, how to use them, and eventually developing a website just to share with anyone who would listen. The next phase came with companies that have outdoor workers and training their safety directors the best practices I had learned about tick prevention. After that came speaking on tick prevention at safety conferences across the country.

With 3-400,000 new Lyme disease cases each year in the US alone, it is a monumental task to bring more awareness and education to the public. Ticks like mosquitos are not going away anytime soon. So we need to know more about how to keep them off from us and what to do if we get bit.

This book has been a joy to write because it allows me to go into a lot of detail while trying to make it fun to read at the same time. I always like to say if you can laugh and learn it makes the learning more fun.

So, keep in mind, it's a war out there that will never go away. I pray the following pages will help you in your battle plan as you enjoy God's beautiful creation, we call earth. Let's make it as tick-free as possible, so read on!

Chapter 1

How I Got Started

Like most people who have unique careers, their child-hood quite often plays a part in their original interest. I am no different in that respect from my fascination with ticks beginning very early as a young boy. It may have taken me several decades for that interest to mature, but here it is none the less.

My story begins in St. Ignace, Michigan, where I was born and spent my first couple years there, then moving south to Blissfield to spend my K-8th grade years. During that time, my family would frequently make the long 500-mile trip to the Upper Peninsula to visit my grandparents in Quinnesec. My grandparents lived in a beautiful country farm location that reminded most people of a quaint little story book setting. To me, the trip to the farm was always a special time of visiting with grandparents, watching different cartoons, enjoying the woods, playing in the barn with cousins, and experiencing the strange little critters we all call ticks.

You see, I didn't have ticks back home, so it was almost a novelty and kinda fun in a weird sort of way. I was very familiar with the pesky mosquito that would land on me, then I would normally feel their bite. The tick was different because most of the time I never even knew when I had one on me until my mom did a tick check just before a bath or bed. If she did find one on me, it was kind of cool because it was like a little skin tag that needed to be pulled off, and that was it. In those days, we never had any problems with ticks, never talked about tick-borne diseases. They were just a minor annoyance, like a mosquito.

So, the days spent at the farm were fun playing and occasionally watching grandpa take ticks off the dog that were sometimes the size of a dime. I am not sure if my brothers and I ever did the hammer test with those big fat ticks, but we may have. However, just for fun I do remember looking for them on blades of grass and occasionally finding them "questing", waiting for their next victim.

Fast forward a few years. I married my high school sweetheart, and we made our first home in the house where my grandparents had once lived. They had passed away, so this beautiful spot in the woods needed some temporary tenants for a few years before my parents would take over the family homestead for their retirement.

To me it was a dream come true, living in the woods, but to my wife it was a culture shock in every sense of the word. She was a trooper and took it in stride pretty well given the circumstances, as I had to introduce her to many new things in rural living. The biggest adjustment for her was the lack of good shopping. This was especially true in the late seventies. Other adjustments were the wild animals like raccoons, woodchucks, coyote, deer, and bears that roamed the nearby woods.

I remember the first time she noticed ticks. It was a nice sunny day, and we decided to have a picnic lunch out in the field just for a change of pace. It was a perfect spot by the edge of the woods that gave us a little shade from the hot sun as we had our lunch. After the meal, I remember thinking how we were the only ones on this 175-acre spot and totally alone. So, as I was gazing at my gorgeous new bride, I decide to try to get a little romance going. Just as things were starting to move in the right direction, she utters those dreaded words "honey what are those little brown things crawling on the blanket?" Of course, my response was "don't worry about those right now." Well, as it turned out, she did worry about those little brown things and that was the end of the "blanket party" in the field that day. However, when we did return to the house, we were able to pick up where we left off by giving her the first lesson of the all-important "tick check." I felt it was very important to be sure that we had no unwelcome little brown things on us.

Fast forward a few more years and along came two kids. By this time, my parents had retired and moved back to the farm, so we moved into town as was originally planned. The kids would often visit the grandparents and grandma wanted to get them used to the woods and the ticks, so she devised a plan. She figured if she would pay the grandkids $.25 cents per tick, it would lessen any fear that they might have of them. Well, it didn't work very well for my daughter because she was very afraid of the ticks no matter what. But my son was a different story. He was a born outdoorsman, an entrepreneur, and loved the idea. He figured if grandma was going to pay him for getting ticks, he was going to make some money on the deal. His first day, he made a dollar from getting four ticks. He was also learning some of the places where he could roll in the grass to pick up more and thus make more money. It didn't take grandma long to figure what was going on, so she had to drop the prize money down to $.10 cents per tick and eventually scrap the whole program before going broke.

Fast forward a few more years when I was doing some residential telephone and satellite wiring. One night I came home from doing some wiring in a crawl space and I felt a "splinter" on my back by my shoulder blade. It was in a very awkward spot where I couldn't reach it, so I asked my wife for some help. I remember asking her to get a needle so she could dig it out. As she was getting ready to poke the needle in and start the extraction suddenly, she gasped and took a step back and said, "there are legs coming out, it's not a sliver, it's a tick." This tick had uncharacteristically buried about half of itself into my back and was not going to come out easily. We then started attempting all the "old wives' tales" in hopes of a simple solution, but no such luck. We tried fingernail polish remover, Vaseline, a match, etc. trying to get the tick to back out, but nothing worked. The next step was to take it to the people I knew who had a lot of experience with ticks and that was my parents.

They lived at the farm where they picked ticks off of themselves, along with their dog, on a daily basis. On one occasion, when they had been out picking raspberries on a two-rut road in the woods, they ended up setting a record for ticks on a dog. That night when they checked over the dog, they had a new farm record, yes 163 ticks that day! Wow that's a lot of ticks. As was customary to them, they would collect all the ticks in a little styrofoam cup and then zap them in the microwave. That night, I'm sure they had to do that several times just because of the sheer number of ticks, but that's how it goes.

Now, since they were such "tick experts" I figured they would know how to remove this tick that was so badly stuck in my back. Believe it or not, they had never seen one stuck quite this bad, so this tick even had them stumped as to the best way to get it out. I had gotten lots of ticks stuck to me over the years and they normally just flopped back and forth like a little skin tag, and they came out easily, but not this one. Well then, the final step was to see a doctor, and that's what I did. I just wanted it out the best way so it would not cause any more problems. So, I saw a doctor, and he forced his fine tipper tweezers down in there and out came the tick. That's pretty much how that one ended and luckily no problems after that.

Fast forward a few more years and one night my wife said, "Honey, you have got to see this Facebook picture." Now you know how sometimes you look at a picture and because it is magnified, you are not quite sure what you are even looking at? This picture was one of those. So,

I ask my wife "I give up what is it?" She said, "it is the white of someone's eyeball and the little brown speck that is circled is a tick stuck to his eye!" Ohhh wow that gives my chills just thinking about it and I felt terrible for the poor guy. Well, as you can imagine, this face book post really got me curious as to all the details of what actually happened. So, then I started researching the story and the next day I called the power company and talked to the safety director who actually posted it on Facebook. He told me that one of their linemen was out on a routine job and in the process of moving some brush out of the way, some "dust" happened to get in his eye. He went on to say that the guy was wearing safety glasses and apparently was doing everything correctly and then noticed what felt like a speck of dust go in his eye.

Once they arrived back at the shop, they began washing it out just like they were supposed to do and nothing would come loose. Needless to say, they were somewhat baffled because the eye wash procedure normally always worked, especially on a little piece of "dust." For some reason, this was a tough one. After a time of trying, they eventually decided that to get some professional help, so they took him to the eye doctor. Once there, it did not take long to get to the bottom of the problem. With all the proper equipment and expert training, the doctor told him to his surprise that he had a baby tick stuck to his eyeball. The next step was to remove it and they say as he was pulling it out with fine tipped tweezers you could hear a "pop" when it actually came out!

What a crazy true story, but we need to always keep in mind that ticks can attach to us any place where there is skin, yes ladies and men... down there too! So, during tick season, it is very important to do daily tick checks in front of a mirror and then shower hopefully in order to wash off any that may not be attached.

More on prevention in a later chapter.

Chapter 2

How Big is the Problem?

The CDC estimates there are at least 300,000 new Lyme disease cases each year in The United States. To put that into perspective, "that's 6 times more than the annual incidence of HIV/AIDS and about 1 1/2 times the number of incidence of breast cancer." (1) When compared with some of these other well-known diseases, it becomes clearer that Lyme disease is really a problem. See below a CDC Lyme disease map from just a few years ago. (2)

"Lyme disease diagnoses have increased dramatically in the US during the past 15 years, rising 357% in rural areas, according to Fair Health." (3)

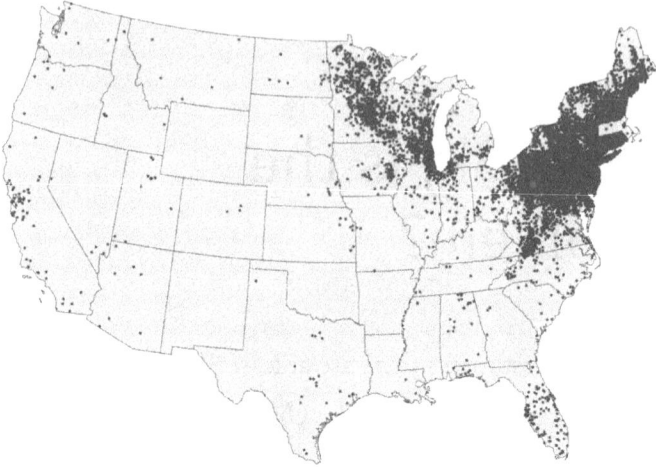

(2)

So, to say there is a problem is an understatement. This is only referring to Lyme, not to mention Anaplasmosis, Babesiosis, Ehrlichiosis, Rocky Mountain Spotted Fever, Powassan Virus (no known cures), and Alpha-gal syndrome (allergy to red meat). Any one of these can be a real pain, life altering, and sometimes even fatal.

Lyme seems to be the biggest and most widespread problem of them all and various reports have said that it has been around for maybe hundreds of years. In the mid-seventies, there were several adolescent kids in a small Connecticut town who were all experiencing some strange symptoms. Thanks to the mothers who pushed the medical community to come up with some answers to their kids' achy joints, flu-like symptoms, unusual fatigue, brain fog, etc. This was the start of what we now call Lyme disease, named after the city of Lyme CT.

It has been widely reported that the number of ticks and their diseases have been on the rise in recent years, with no signs of letting up. Reports have noted a few things that could be contributing to the steady increase.

Things like more rural living, which in turn naturally put more people in tick habitat, therefore more opportunity to get tick bites, and there are more outdoor adventure seeking types of people too. Those include groups like hikers, meaning day hikers who pack a lunch and head out for several hours and hike normally less than 10 miles.

Then you have the more serious hikers we call backpackers because they will go out for days, weeks, and months at a time. Rustic camping in tents is very popular in somewhat remote areas as well.

Exploring straight through the woods looking for mushrooms and deer sheds (antlers) in the spring is also common and makes one very susceptible to picking up ticks during the worst time of the year. Our society is just more mobile than past generations, putting us in tick habitats more often, and making us easy targets for those little blood suckers. This can also help spread them to new areas when we bring them home and also puts us in danger of getting bitten.

Birds, by their nature, will also carry ticks to new locations as they migrate to help spread tick numbers even further. Don't forget the ever-popular white-tail deer that generally has strong numbers across the country. The deer are a prime host for ticks where they frequently feed and then breed all the while on the deer for their final season.

Climate change can also contribute to ticks numbers, as they prefer warmer weather conditions, which help them thrive better. Popular thinking has been that because of the warmer temperatures, springtime has been coming earlier and winter has been later. With this thought, ticks have been given more time to look for a host and when finding one, their life can be extended even further.

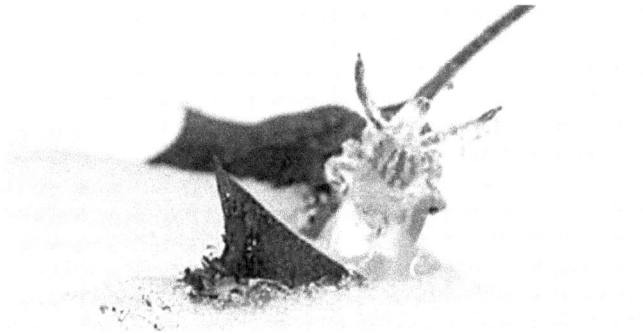

(4)

Ticks almost never freeze to death because during the winter months in colder climates they will dive under the leaf litter for their dormant season. They were also created with a special God given liquid that acts as an antifreeze to aid them during those harsh cold months. In addition, they take full advantage of being under the snow, which is also a great insulator. Experts say that 32-40 degrees is about the temperature when ticks seem to go down for the winter and when they come out in the spring. It is not uncommon for ticks to reappear temporarily during those warm days in a January or February thaw. This is in the northern states, so keep in mind tick activity will vary based on the weather that they live in. Yes, we are all disappointed that the winter does not kill them off like we hoped it would, but that's the way it is. In most warmer climate states, tick activity slows down a lot but never entirely to a complete standstill.

The bottom line is that ticks are a very hardy pest, and they are not going away any time soon. We just need to somehow coexist with them and learn to avoid them, just like we do with the pesky mosquito.

The purpose of this book is to help you learn more about the enemy (ticks) because it is a war out there. The more you know about this enemy the better you can avoid them, repel them, remove them, terminate them, and if bitten know what to do next. We cannot allow them to win and keep us inside because we are smarter than they are and we want to still be able to enjoy the beautiful woods God created for us.

Chapter 3

Know Your Enemy

As you can see on the banner below, our geniously designed logo is a tick in the shape of a hand grenade. I never knew I could have so much fun with a logo, but it fits perfectly with what I do. The reason I enjoy it so much is that it really is a war out there against ticks. I like to think that any good military leader must study and know his enemy if he wants to be successful in battle. Well, that is exactly what I have done for a number of years and I'm still learning about those darn little blood suckers almost every day. This book is to help you learn too, so here we go.

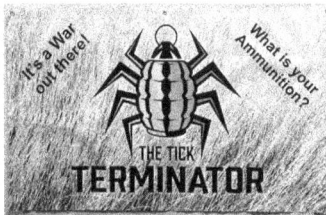

Did you know that there are over 800 tick species in the world? Yes, they are all over the place, not just here in the US or wherever you live. However, the vast majority of them do not bite humans but instead they prey on animals and birds. In the US, we have several dozen ticks species but only about a dozen give us any problems. I wish they were not so widespread but that's just in fairy tales.

I am not going to get into all the fancy scientific names and sound like a I have PhD in entomology because I don't. I like to keep things simple and straight forward and try to make it fun to learn about such an annoying little creature.

For starters, the tick is part of the spider family, so they are actually arachnids. Most people think they are insects, so next time you are discussing ticks at a dinner party, you can impress your friends by telling them that ticks are indeed arachnids, and they will be blown away with your knowledge.

Ticks in the US are broken down into two categories: soft body and hard body. The hard body ticks have the biggest numbers by far, so that in turn makes them the biggest problem too.

The "soft tick" is generally found in the south and western part of the US and will normally be found living in rodent nests of old abandoned buildings, cabins or just unkept dwellings. They are very sneaky and if someone decides to sleep in their area, these ticks may come down from their nest and feed on the unsuspecting house guest during the night. The tick will only feed for a short time (maybe 30 minutes) then return its nest.

The sad thing is the person does not even know what happened until they start to feel sick in the coming days with maybe "tick borne relapsing fever." Common symptoms are high fever, headaches, and achy muscles and joints. Best course of action is to see a doctor very soon because treatment with antibiotics will usually take care of it. Moral of this short story is don't sleep in old, abandoned mountain cabins or trapper shacks, etc. You never know what can happen when you are asleep.

The "hard tick" is the most common tick in the US and because of that, we will spend the most time on them. See the following pages and pics of the "Big Three" yes, the ones that cause the most problems for all of us.

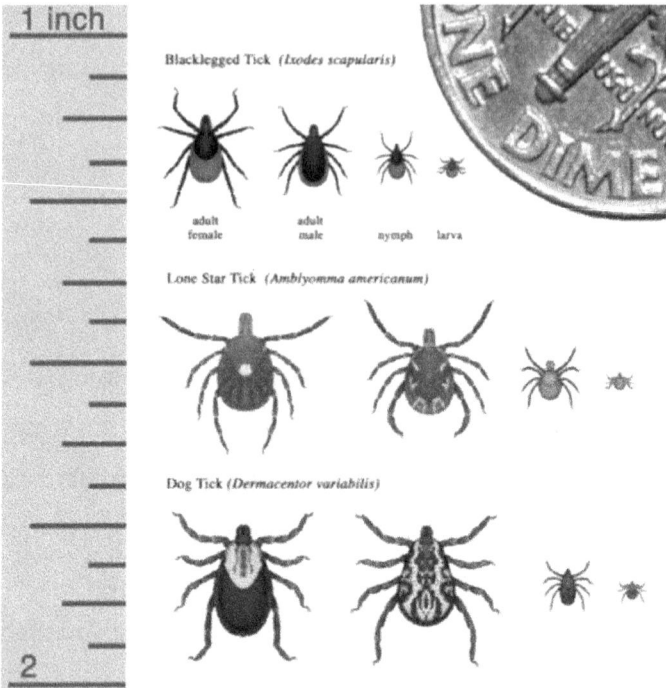

Diagram by the CDC (1)

The ticks are displayed with the female as the larger of the two adults. Note the female is also the one who most likely will be found feeding on humans, as the male rarely feeds on humans.

The life cycle is a big mystery to most people, and they are normally quite intrigued when I explain it to them.

It starts off when the female gives birth to anywhere between 1000 to 5000 eggs in spring or early summer.

After about two weeks, the eggs start to hatch, and new baby ticks are born. Yes, I know that is a lot of eggs and I wish it was only like fifty, but it really is in the thousands. So once the eggs hatch, the newborn ticks are now larva and want something just like all newborns want and that is food. Keep in mind most ticks only eat one time a year and also only have one thing on their menu, and that's blood. At this stage in their life, the larva is just a speck on the forest floor and are not very mobile, so their first meal has to be something very close to the ground as well. Since the options are very limited, the first opportunity for their food is often the normal every day white-footed mouse.

They get on the mouse and go right for a meal and start sucking the blood to satisfy their newborn hunger. In the process, they may take in some bad pathogens (germs) from the mouse, and this is where the trouble begins. You see, ticks are not born with any diseases. They normally pick them up from their first host (the mouse) and then they will carry them for the rest of their lives. After about 3 days of feasting on the mouse, they drop off and bask in a delightful feeling of a full belly, or should I say, full body. Next, they do nothing during the fall and winter as they snuggle down in the leaf litter and molt into the nymph stage.

When they come back to normal activity the following spring, they have grown two more legs (born with 6 now have 8) and will be the size of a poppy seed. This nymph stage is a dangerous stage to us humans because they are so small, we can barely see them on our shoelaces, let alone anywhere else. Remember, if they picked up Lyme or any other tick-borne disease (they can carry more than one) from their first host, they can now pass it along to their next host. A large percentage of people who get Lyme and other tick-borne diseases get it from the nymph stage ticks because they are so small, they can go unnoticed until it's too late. The nymph ticks generally feed for about 3 days, then drop off, enjoy their meal, molt into the adult size during the fall and winter down under the leaf litter, and then wait for spring.

As an adult, they will look for another host for their annual blood meal, which can again be us, some other animal. Quite often it is a deer. Once on the deer, the male and female will feed, mate, and stay on their final host until the next spring. When spring comes, the male drops off and dies and the female drops off and gives birth to several thousand tick eggs. That's enough to kill anyone, so she dies too.

To recap the life cycle of a tick, it is born an egg, molts into the larva, then the nymph, and finally the adult tick. They eat once a year and live for about 3 years. If they cannot find a host on one of those years they are naturally terminated.

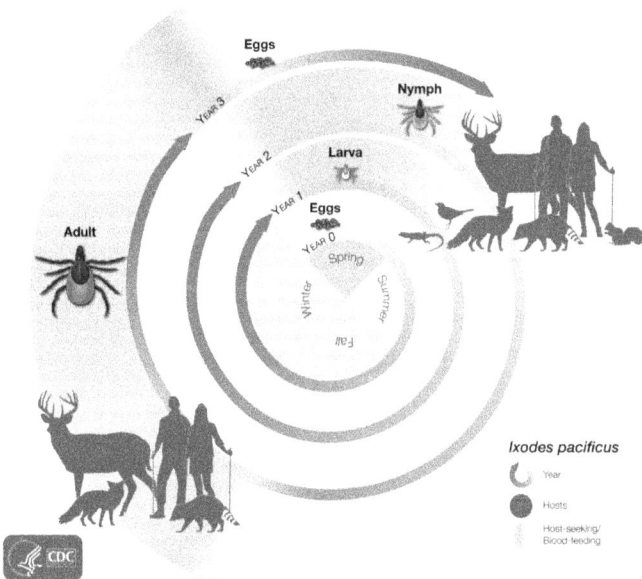

This diagram shows the lifecycle of blacklegged ticks that can transmit Lyme disease. Diagram by CDC (2)

Ticks also have natural enemies, like any other creature in the wild. The popular ones are ants, spiders, praying mantis, grasshoppers, centipedes, opossums, nematodes, some birds, and quail to name a few. Also, some domesticated members of the poultry family, like chickens, guinea hens, and turkeys, enjoy eating ticks too. Wild turkeys are really known for liking ticks along with ants, spiders, praying mantis, grasshoppers, all at the same time. They say that turkeys have a voracious appetite when going through the woods and eat all those little bugs that also like to eat ticks. Studies have basically said that turkeys are like pigs with wings in the woods. They eat so many of the natural enemies of the tick that it helps the tick thrive even more because now they have fewer enemies. Who would have ever thought that the darn turkeys could be helping to aid in the rising tick population?

It is very important to do daily tick checks and always use permethrin tick and insect repellant when out in tick habitat.

Speaking of the tick habitat, I want to clear up a few "old wives' tales." Contrary to popular belief, ticks do not fly, jump, run, climb trees, or drop from trees in the USA. Instead, most of them will be found "questing" (sitting) on a blade of grass or some kind of low-lying vegetation. They just sit there patiently waiting with their two outstretched legs for a host so they can latch on as it brushes by.

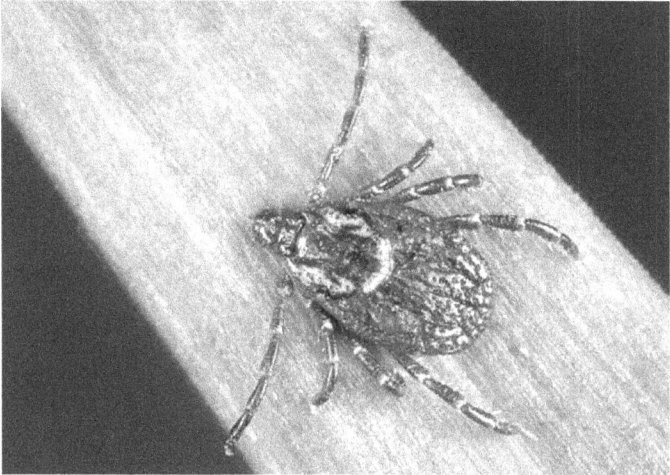

Picture by CDC (3)

Once on their newfound host, they crawl around, looking for a nice place to start their meal. They generally end up behind the knee, waistline, hairline behind the ears, and any place where there is skin. See the diagram on the following page for those "meal" places. I like to say they are very rude hitchhikers who don't even ask permission but just attach to whoever and whatever, then go for their blood.

They are going to prefer a moist area if at all possible because they need the moisture to survive. That's why they are so often found in tall grass and knee-high vegetation.

As an example, you would never find a tick out in the middle of a parking lot because there is no protection there for them and it's way too hot.

5 Tick Prevention Methods to also consider:

1. Tuck your pants into your socks. This will keep the ticks on the outside and if your pants are treated with permethrin, it will drive them crazy and eventually be their demise—Yaaaa

2. Wear light-colored clothes so ticks are easy to spot if they get on you.

3. Walk on well-used paths away from any vegetation.

4. Use 25-35% Deet on exposed skin.

5. Treat your shoes, socks, pants, and shirts with permethrin.

Protect Yourself Against Lyme Disease
Any time the Temps rise above 35F

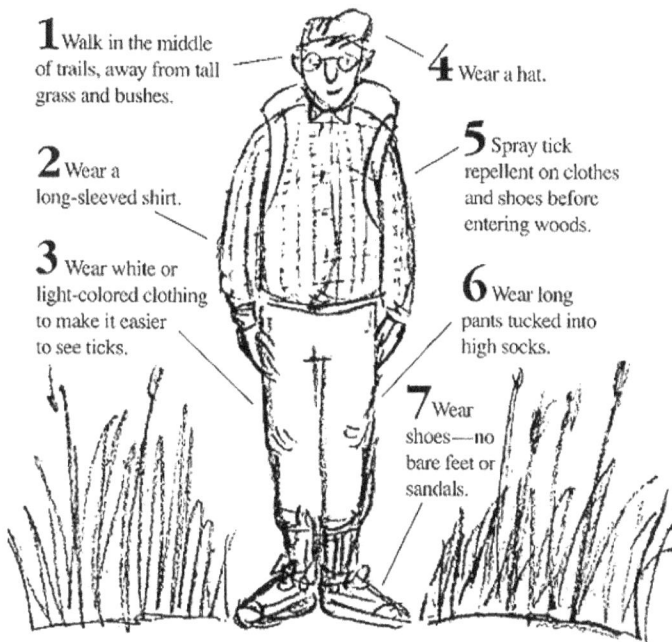

1 Walk in the middle of trails, away from tall grass and bushes.

2 Wear a long-sleeved shirt.

3 Wear white or light-colored clothing to make it easier to see ticks.

4 Wear a hat.

5 Spray tick repellent on clothes and shoes before entering woods.

6 Wear long pants tucked into high socks.

7 Wear shoes—no bare feet or sandals.

Drawing from www.lymeticks.org (4)

When you get home and are doing your tick check, *if* you notice a tick on your clothes, keep in mind where there's one, there may be more. See "below" diagram for the most common places to look.

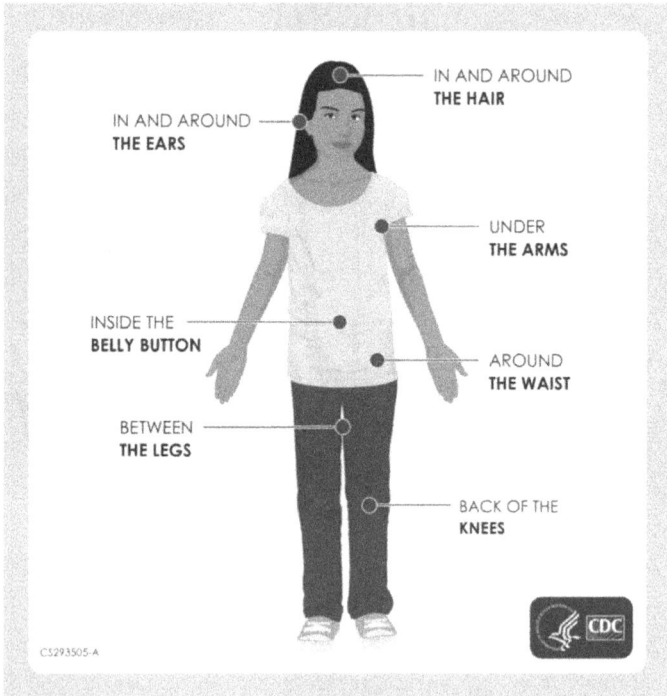

Diagram by CDC (5)

Here is a little-known trick: take all your clothes and throw them into the dryer (not the washer) on high for about 15 minutes. The dry heat is really hard on ticks and it will kill them. After that, then you can throw them in the washer. As a rule, ticks don't normally last in a house much more than a few days anyway because it is too dry for them. The dryer trick just makes sure they are terminated before they even have a chance to attach to anyone and cause problems.

During some of my early research about 10 years ago, I was trying to learn how ticks would react to various smells, scents, and odors. It was painstaking to try to figure them out as I would place them on the white carpet in our basement. The grandkids called it "woodticking with papa" as we proceeded to make many trips upstairs to find a variety of cleaning products, food, etc. just to see if they would react in any way on the carpet. At that time, one of my goals was to try to figure out what their "chocolate" or some favorite flavor of something that they would find more appealing than our blood. Well, I did find out that our blood is number #1 and nothing comes very close. During that process, I did learn a few interesting smells and odors that they do and don't like, mostly from research online.

I found that they don't like:

- essential oils

- peppermint

- lemon

- eucalyptus

- lavender

- cedar

- citronella

- vinegar

- citrus

Some people use these products for their own tick repellants with limited results, but one guy I met has a whole new twist on the subject.

A few years ago, I was doing a video segment on tick prevention with Larry Smith from Larry Smith Outdoors. As usual, we were laughing and joking around, and when I brought up the topic of smells that ticks don't like and when I mentioned citrus, he just stopped and said, "they don't like citrus?" I assured him that no; they didn't. He then started to tell me that for some reason he never seems to be bothered by ticks (I told him count his blessings). He knows a few friends that have had real problems with Lyme disease, but he has managed to avoid it for some reason. He then tells me that he just loves Sun Drop soda (citrus flavor) and drinks about 6 bottles a day. I looked at him and broke out in a big grin and said, "Holy smokes, you drink so much of that stuff it's probably coming out of your pores." To top it off, ticks probably can smell you coming and to them you stink like a disgusting sewer. It's no wonder you never get bit." Now, to be honest, I'm not sure if that is actually the case, but who knows, it could be a factor. If nothing else, we sure had a good laugh over it.

Like most living creatures, ticks have smells they really take a liking to. They love the smell of:

- Moisture

- Sweaty smells

- CO_2 we breathe out

- Urine

- Anything else that may remind them of mammals.

They have to rely heavily on their sense of smell, vibrations, and even sensing body heat from their potential host. The reason is that most of them have very poor eyesight and in some species none at all.

So, the million dollar question is, how do we get rid of them or at least keep them away from us? Well, I don't think we will ever eliminate them completely, but the next chapter will discuss different prevention ideas, methods, and best practices.

Chapter 4

How to Get Rid of Them

I hate to say this again, but those darn disgusting little suckers are pretty much like mosquitos, and they are here to stay. I have also seen and read an awful lot of ideas about how to eliminate or just somehow limit their numbers. So, with that said, I will list a few cool ideas of what is going on out there, but keep in mind this list will continue to grow every year.

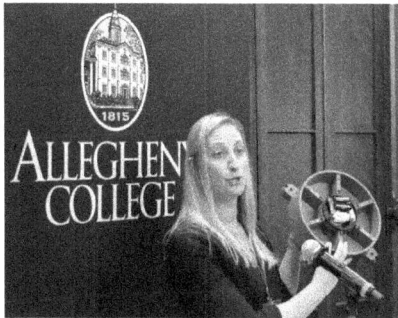

(1)

During a press conference on April 26, 2022, at Allegheny College, Nicole Chinnici, director of the Pennsylvania Tick Research Lab, presented a unique study she has been working on for about five years. Keep in mind that Pennsylvania is one of the top states for Lyme disease in the US, so it is no surprise that a study of this nature would come from there.

The study "will revolve around the vaccination of small mammals, mainly white-footed mice, and its effectiveness in reducing tick population." It will take place in several counties and be quite involved over a period of about 3-5 years to account for the life cycle of ticks and mice.

They developed special bait stations (see the previous page picture) where they will place food pellets treated with a vaccine for the mice to eat."The vaccine works by affecting the saliva of a tick whenever it bites into a vaccinated animal and is similar to treatments given to pets to ward off fleas and ticks. Chinnici said the vaccine cements the saliva of the tick and causes them to fall off. The insect will either die or be prevented from advancing through its lifecycle afterward." (1)

They are hoping the vaccine will cut back on the numbers of ticks, then in turn there will be fewer tick-borne diseases. This study is the first of its kind in the US and I wish them the best.

Another study that was talked about several years ago puts an unusual twist with mice that is very different from the previous story.

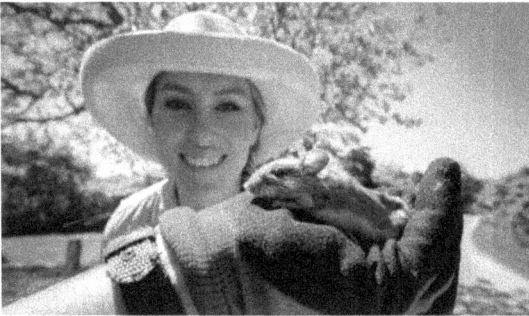

(2)

This creative—or as some would say, "radical" idea is to "engineer mice and stop Lyme disease." Scientists Kevin Esvelt, and Duane Wesemann are proposing to genetically modify a bunch of white-footed mice for Martha's Vineyard and Nantucket Island in hopes of stopping Lyme disease. The plan is to genetically modify mice then let them loose on the islands to then interbreed with the existing mice that are already on the islands. The idea is that these "new mice" will be altered so that when ticks feed on these mice, the pathogens (germs) that they are sucking out of them will not produce Lyme in the tick.

So, if the tick does not get Lyme from the mice (normally their first host) the theory is that when and if the ticks feed on a human as their second host they will not pass on Lyme to the humans.

The concerns of releasing the proposed 100k plus mice on these islands and what it will do to the environment is anyone's guess at this point. However, I hope that their testing plans will be successful on some uninhabited island, so they might do the real thing where it will help a lot of people. (2)

We have all heard of exterminators who will go to a business or residence and help get rid of all sorts of bugs. They are known for removing cockroaches, ants, ticks, mosquitos, and almost any other type of pesky bugs.

Now there is a private company that goes even further than that. I mean, they will help control ticks, mosquitos, and even poison ivy on an even larger scale.

See the following info on ticks from their website.

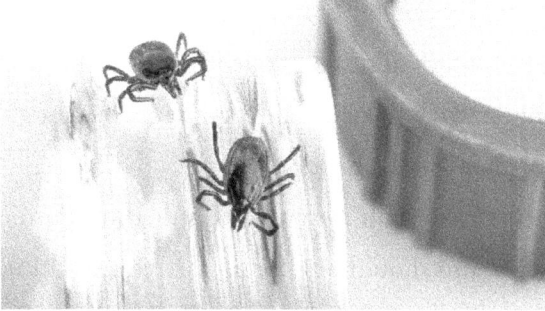

(3)

"Our Tick Population Analysis service will provide you with a detailed understanding of the tick population levels, distribution and disease infection rate. This analysis is completed through Ivy Oaks Analytics and our University Laboratory partner. This service is available to county governments, military bases, neighborhoods, summer camps, academic campuses, large estates, resorts, farms and similar entities."

Sounds like a great idea and some good peace for mom when she sends Johnny and Susie off to summer camp.

They are currently operating mostly in the eastern half of the United States. (3)

Yet another way to try to eliminate those darn ticks is something I have actually heard of and have also been asked about on several occasions. This method involves "heat" and I mean lots of it, in other words kill them with fire! Some may call it controlled burning or prescribed burning, anyway you slice it if you give them enough heat. They are going to be history.

I want to say right now that this method can be very dangerous and should only be used after consulting with local fire professionals, forestry personnel, and maybe even the DNR.

One interesting study was done over a several-year span by Elizabeth Gleim, a graduate student at the Warnell School of Forestry and Natural Resources. "During that time, she visited 21 plots in Georgia and Florida to collect tick samples monthly. Most of those plots had been subjected to long-term prescribed burning, a way to manage and control the growth of plant and animal species on a specific area of land."

Her findings were quite interesting.

She found the prescribed burning over a long period of time effectively reduced tick populations and changed the landscape of the burned area.

She says, "At the end of the day, prescribed fire on a long-term basis decimated tick population, it's exciting because by reducing tick populations, the technique indicated that it was reducing risk of tick-borne disease in humans while also enhancing ecosystem health."

She noted that on the plots where there was no burning, the tick counts were 10 times greater than the burned sites.

In total, over 47,000 ticks were collected among the 21 sites over two years. She also stressed to do prompt tick checks after visiting the forest and to use Deet or permethrin repellants to help keep ticks off. "UGA research links prescribed burning to reduce tick populations." (4)

Dry Ice tick traps—like the following picture shows it is normally a do-it-yourself project.

This is a very basic device that could be made mostly with just stuff around the house and the garage. All you really need is a container like an old plastic cooler or Styrofoam cooler, a chunk of plywood, some double-sided sticky back tape, then get some dry ice.

Next, cut the plywood so you can put your container in the middle of it. Be sure to leave space to put the double-sided sticky back tape all around the cooler like in the picture. Then, put a hole (one inch diameter at the most) in each side of the container. Next, get some dry ice and be sure to use gloves and put some in the container and close the lid.

As the dry ice starts to melt, it will escape through the holes and it will smell like CO_2 to any nearby ticks. They will notice the smell because it smells like what we breathe out and they will come toward the smell. When they get close enough, they will get stuck on the tape and now you "got 'em."

Keep in mind the dry ice will need to be replaced, so check it often because this method requires some attention.

Well, there you have it a cheap homemade idea for a garden area, backyard, or small play area to help cut down on the tick population.

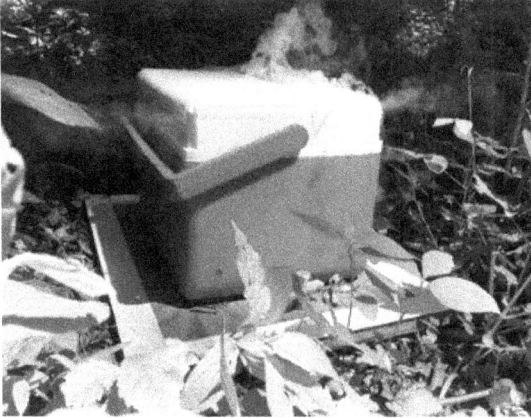

Credit Solny Adalsteinsson - This is a baited tick trap containing carbon dioxide-producing dry ice. The lone star tick is an active hunter, following trails of carbon dioxide to sniff out hosts up to 16 feet away. (5)

The Tick Tube is another way of helping to drop the number of ticks in your yard. This is one I have actually done several times for my parent's yard in the country, and I think it has helped a little. The tick tubes can be bought online or made easily for almost nothing. I even have them listed on my website as an example of a type of "tick deterrent." They are basically the core of a toilet paper roll with permethrin treated cotton balls stuffed inside. See the following picture of how it plays out.

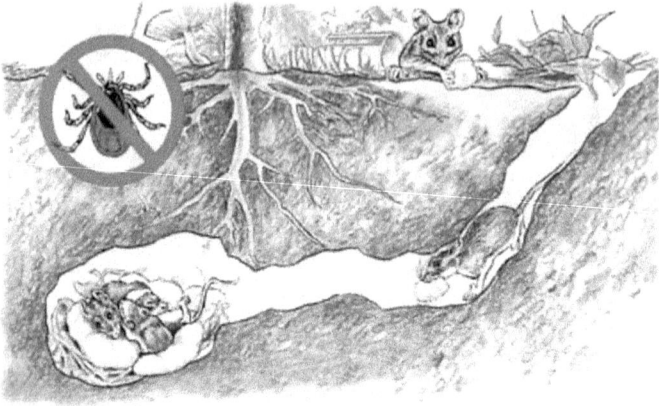

(6)

In the picture (Damminix tick tubes) the mouse up on ground level notices the toilet paper tube that has been placed around the yard in his territory with nice little cotton balls stuffed inside. He says "Wow look at these nice cotton balls, they will work great for bedding down in my underground home." So he steals them right out of the tubes and takes them home to show Mrs. Mouse. She loves them too, so they use them for extra bedding and they work out very well.

The next part of the theory is that the "newborn" ticks will usually get on mice as their first host (meal) because they are born on the ground and mice are very accessible to them. Once on the mice, they will generally feed for a few days and then drop off during the daytime hours. This is a good thing because mice are normally sleeping during the day, so when the baby ticks drop off, the idea is that they will land right into the permethrin treated cotton balls. At this point, the treated cotton goes to work on their delicate little bodies and soon after that, they are dead. The best part about this is they are terminated before they ever reach any humans, yaaaa.

Two of the popular names who sell the tick tubes already set up and ready to go are Damminix and Thermacell.

Some people who live in heavy tick habitat areas will also try to tick proof their own yard. See below info and diagram for your own ideas by CT Ag Exp Station.

- Remove leaf litter.

- Clear tall grasses and brush around homes and at the edge of lawns.

- Place a 3-ft wide barrier of wood chips or gravel between lawns and wooded areas to restrict tick migration into recreational areas.

- Mow the lawn frequently.

- Stack wood neatly and in a dry area (discourages rodents).

- Keep playground equipment, decks, and patios away from yard edges and trees.

- Discourage unwelcome animals (such as deer, raccoons, and stray dogs) from entering your yard by constructing fences.

- Remove old furniture, mattresses, or trash from the yard that may give ticks a place to hide. (7)

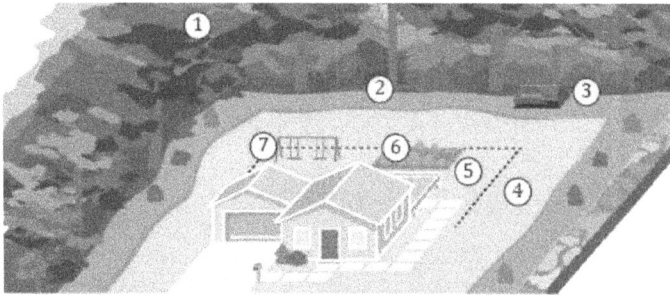

1	Tick zone	Avoid areas with forest and brush where deer, rodents, and ticks are common.
2	Wood chip barrier	Use a 3 ft. barrier of wood chips or rock to separate the "tick zone" and rock walls from the lawn.
3	Wood pile	Keep wood piles on the wood chip barrier, away from the home.
4	Tick migration zone	Maintain a 9 ft. barrier of lawn between the wood chips and areas such as patios, gardens, and play sets.
5	Tick safe zone	Enjoy daily living activities such as gardening and outdoor play inside this perimeter.
6	Gardens	Plant deer resistant crops. If desired, an 8-ft. fence can keep deer out of the yard.
7	Play sets	Keep play sets in the "tick safe zone" in sunny areas where ticks have difficulty surviving.

Based on a diagram by K. Stafford, Connecticut Agricultural Experiment Station

(8)

In the next chapter, I will discuss the most popular personal repellants.

Chapter 5

Personal Bug Repellants

This is one of my favorite topics and I hope you will learn something for your own personal protection and use it the next time you are in the woods or in your own backyard. Let me say right at the beginning, all "bug" repellants are not created equal, some are natural and some are synthetic. Some are for your skin, some are for your clothes and gear, some will last for 1-2 hours, 12 hours, a couple days, several months, and some will last for a couple of years.

There are also some other types of "tick deterrents" that give a wide variety of results. Some use permethrin treated gaiters on their shins (see next page), light-colored clothes to spot them, duct tape pants to their boots so ticks can't crawl up their legs, use lint rollers and full-length mirrors for tick checks at home, and still others will try scented soaps and shampoos to keep the bugs away.

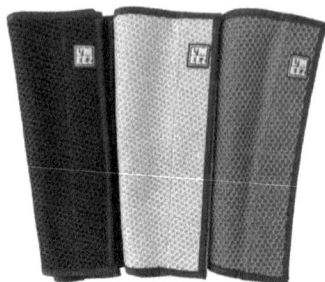

(1)

About twenty years ago, they tried a vaccine for Lyme disease but had some problems and had to discontinue it. At the moment, there are still no vaccines, and even if there were, it would be hard to get one to work against all the tick-borne diseases out there. The big problem is that Lyme and other tick-borne diseases respond so differently in different people. It seems each case almost needs special treatment, especially when they have been sick for many months. So, the best thing for prevention is still using some kind of repellant.

Obviously, the choice will be yours, so I will just talk about some of the most popular options that are available on the market. Your selections will vary based on your needs. Some things to consider when looking at repellants is how and what you will use them for?

- Gardening in the backyard?

- A casual 1-3 mile hike on the weekend?

- All day long for an outdoor worker?

- A three week backpacking trip?

- Three-month hunting season?

With those thoughts, let's review some of the choices that you will have.

Repellants are available in several forms, to fit almost any application. You should always use repellants that are EPA registered and then use as directed. Here are some popular options:

- Lotions to be applied with your hands.

- Aerosols for skin and clothes.

- Towelette or wipes for skin.

- Water borne pump sprays for skin and clothes.

- Concentrates for custom mixing and longer protection.

- Clothes with repellants impregnated into the fabric.

Repellants also come in numerous sizes of application containers to fit almost any need. Here are a few:

- 2-20oz lotions.

- 4-18oz aerosols.

- Individually packaged towelettes.

- 6-128oz (1-gallon) water borne pump sprays.

- 8oz concentrates for mixing.

How do most bug repellants actually work??? Well, glad you asked because here are some of the answers in regular terms. I will skip the scientific verbiage because it confuses me too (you are welcome).

Most of them work based on their scent, smell, or odor that they give off. Let's say you have a mosquito flying around you, looking for a nice spot to land and suck some of your tasty blood. All of a sudden, their little sensory antennas notice this smell on you that doesn't quite seem right. Now keep in mind the smell of the repellant was especially designed to confuse that pesky little blood sucker. What it does is the smell talks to their puny little brain and gives them confusing mixed messages and tells them there is no blood there. Because of that, they fly off and you are the winner because they did not have you for lunch. Yaaa for you! Good job for using an effective bug repellant. So, what are good bug repellants, very good question.

The "big 4" bug repellants are generally thought to be the following based on effectiveness, availability, and popularity:

- Deet

- Picardin

- IR3535

- Oil of lemon eucalyptus

Deet is by far without question the most popular and is used in all kinds of repellants as the active ingredient. It was created in about 1944 for the US Army and later on it became available for civilians in 1957.(2) About the only downside is it can damage some plastics and synthetic fabrics, but it is considered okay to use on natural fabrics. So its primary use is for skin and natural fabrics. Note that "This repellant has been subjected to more scientific and toxicologic scrutiny than any other repellant substance. Deet has a remarkable safety record after 40 years of use and nearly 8 billion human applications."(3)

Most people don't even realize they are using Deet, they just look for the brand name they like and know it's going to work. Another interesting thing most people don't know is what is the difference between lower percentage rate like the 20% vs 100% Deet? People just assume that the 100% has to be stronger, but the biggest difference is that it will just plain last longer. In the majority of cases, 20-30% is the preferred level which can last around 3-6 hours, the 100% can last past 10 hours before needing to reapply.

Assorted sizes are available in:

- Pump spray

- Aerosol

- Towelette / wipes

- Lotion / cream

The next repellant is **Picaridin**. According to Wikipedia:

"**Icaridin**, also known as **picaridin**, is an insect repellent which can be used directly on skin or clothing. It has broad efficacy against various arthropods such as mosquitos, ticks, gnats, flies and fleas, and is almost colorless and odorless. A study performed in 2010 showed that picaridin spray and cream at the 20% concentration provided 12 hours of protection against ticks. Icaridin does not dissolve plastics, synthetics or sealants.

The name *picaridin* was proposed as an International Nonproprietary Name (INN) to the World Health Organization (WHO), but the official name that has been approved by the WHO is *icaridin*.

The chemical is part of the piperidine family, along with many pharmaceuticals and alkaloids such as piperine, which gives black pepper its spicy taste.

Trade names include **Bayrepel** and **Saltidin** among others. The compound was developed by the German chemical company Bayer and was given the name *Bayrepel*. In 2005, Lanxess AG and its subsidiary Saltigo GmbH were spun off from Bayer and the product was renamed *Saltidin* in 2008.

On 23 July 2020, icaridin was approved again by the EU Commission for use in repellent products. The approval entered into force on 1 February 2022 and is valid for ten years." (4)

Picaridin is relatively new compared to Deet and comes in a few different versions, but the 20% mixture is the standard preferred level for best results.

Popular application options are as follows:

- Pump sprays.

- Aerosol.

- Towelette wipes.

- Lotions / creams.

IR3535, is a little lesser known, but don't let that make you think it is any less effective because that would be wrong.

It has a very long scientific name, so it is no wonder they call it IR3535 for short. Wikipedia's definition is:

"Ethyl butylacetylaminopropionate (trade name **IR3535**) is an insect repellent which is applied topically to prevent bites and stings from mosquitos, ticks, and other insects. It is a colorless and almost odorless oil, has efficacy against a broad range of insects, and is reasonably biodegradable." Info taken from Wikipedia.

The Merck website, producer of IR3535®, says, "We developed the insect repellent IR3535® **more than 30 years ago**. Since then, it has become an established ingredient for protecting you and your family against mosquitoes, ticks, and other bugs. Whether you're playing sports, exploring lakes or jungles, canoeing on a river, or just relaxing on a beach watching the sunset, IR3535® will protect you for hours. But one of the best things about IR3535® is that **it shields you without harming** your health or the environment. As a result, it is already well known in many countries as a highly reliable and tolerable repelling agent against ticks, mosquitoes, and other irritating insects, such as head lice."

IR3535® has been successfully used in insect repellents for over 30 years. And how can we prove that it really does what we state? By pointing to a variety of field and "arm in cage" studies, which confirm that our insect repellent works effectively in repelling different kinds of bugs. According to the World Health Organization (WHO), protection against mosquito bites is key to preventing Zika and other insect-borne diseases. One option is to wear clothes that cover as much of the body as possible. In fact, all kinds of physical barriers are important (such as window screens, doors, and windows). Some people sleep under mosquito nets. And others use insect repellents containing IR3535®, DEET, or Icaridin (also known as Picaridin).

IR3535®'s efficacy is also **confirmed by the recommendations of official bodies** such as the CDC (Centers for Disease Control) and EPA (Environmental Protection

Agency). Thanks to our scientific team, which is always exploring the capabilities of IR3535®, a growing number of brands now use this important ingredient, offering you a **variety of products suitable for all family members**." (6)

This unique repellant is available in the following application choices:

- Lotions

- Sticks

- Towelettes wipes

- Aerosols

- Pump sprays

Oil of Lemon Eucalyptus

This repellant would fall under the more "Natural" based repellants that I talk about, as stated in the following Consumer Reports article by Catherine Roberts 7/21/22.

"For people who prefer a plant-based alternative to deet, OLE offers one reliable option.

Here, we explain what oil of lemon eucalyptus is, how well it performs in our tests, and what you need to know about its safety.

What Is Oil of Lemon Eucalyptus?

Let's start with what OLE isn't: It's not an essential oil, despite a name that would understandably make you think otherwise. Instead, it's refined from oil extracted from the Australian plant Corymbia citriodora, also known as lemon- scented gum. (That's another misleading aspect of the name oil of lemon eucalyptus: Corymbia citriodora used to be considered a member of the Eucalyptus genus, but it isn't anymore.)

The main component of oil of lemon eucalyptus that gives it its repellency to bugs is a chemical called p-Men-

thane-3,8-diol, or PMD. PMD came to the attention of U
.S. scientists in the 1990s, after they learned that a Chinese
insect repellent, called Quwenling, was performing better than many other plant-based repellents. Quwenling's
main component is PMD.

How Well Does OLE Work?

CR tests insect repellents by having volunteers put their
repellent-covered arms into cages full of disease-free mosquitoes and seeing how long it takes for them to start
biting. Our current ratings include eight products we've
tested that have 30 percent oil of lemon eucalyptus. Of
those, four performed well enough to earn our recommen-
dation—which means they provided at least 5 hours of
protection against mosquito bites.

Is Oil of Lemon Eucalyptus Safe?

The safety of OLE isn't as well studied as, for instance,
deet. But evidence suggests that it poses little risk when
used according to the label. For one thing, the EPA classi-
fies oil of lemon eucalyptus as a biopesticide, which means

that it's a naturally occurring substance considered to be a lower risk than more conventional pesticides.

The main risk of oil of lemon eucalyptus is that it could be harmful to your eyes, so take care to avoid spraying it in such a way that it might get in your eyes. As always, when applying repellent to your face, you should spray it into your hands first and rub it onto your face.

The other caveat: Oil of lemon eucalyptus shouldn't be used on young children. "It's not registered for children under 3 years of age," says Mustapha Debboun, PhD, a medical and veterinary entomologist and general manager of the Delta Mosquito & Vector Control District in Visalia, Calif. OLE's safety hasn't been well studied in this group." (7)

FYI for the most part, "natural" based repellants work ok but do not have very long staying power and have to be reapplied more frequently. So if you are the natural type, just keep that in mind. They also commonly have active ingredient scents that ticks and bugs don't like as we discussed in chapter 3.

Here are a few options:
- Essential oils

- Lavender

- Cedar

- Citrus

- Oil of lemon eucalyptus

- Citronella

- Geranium

All these special repellants also come in a variety of sizes and different applicators like most repellants:

- Pump sprays

- Aerosols

- Lotions

Keep in mind there are tons of repellants out there, so whatever repellant you choose to help in your "battle with the bugs" always use as directed.

Another idea I recently learned about that is not a repellant but makes a lot of sense is called "Herbal Prophylaxis."

I ran into this when I was reading a really good book that you should also consider reading entitled "Preventing Lyme & Other Tick-Borne Diseases," by Alexis Chesney. In a nutshell, it means if you are the type of person who is in tick habitat a lot, the thought is to build up your immune system "as a preventative measure" even before you are bitten.

Chapter 4 of the book, Herbal Prophylaxis for Lyme and Tick-Borne Disease has this to say:

"Implementing tick bite prevention strategies is crucial, but equally important is knowing when to administer prophylaxis—that is, "a measure taken to prevent disease." Prophylaxis measures can be initiated by anyone immediately after finding a tick bite, and they can be used regularly by people at high risk for tick bites. This chapter explores the importance of prophylaxis, identifies which herbal formulas can be used as prophylaxis for which types of tick bites, and examines the herbs used to make the formulas."

Why Prophylaxis?

I believe that prophylaxis is important because it can be so difficult to diagnose Lyme and other tick-borne disease (TBD) properly. Prophylaxis allows you to take measures to treat illness preemptively before it even manifests as symptoms in your body. The philosophy is not unique to tick-borne diseases. For example, people who are going to visit regions where malaria is endemic are encouraged to take a prophylaxis pharmaceutical regimen, before they travel, to protect themselves just in case they are bitten by a mosquito that transmits the protozoan that causes malaria. Better to treat ahead of time than wait for symptoms and diagnosis.

The same holds true for Lyme and other TBD. Whether you are bitten by a tick or simply living, working, or recreating in an area where these diseases are endemic, you can take measures to prevent infections with these diseases. My preference for the prophylactic approach is based on several factors regarding Lyme and TBD diagnostics:

Fewer than 50 percent of people with Lyme disease remember receiving a tick bite.

Fewer than 50 percent of people with Lyme disease see a bull's-eye rash.

- Symptoms of Lyme disease may take 30 days or more to develop after a tick bite.

- Conventional Lyme disease and babesiosis testing is not reliable.

- There are no testing options for TBD like those caused by certain *Borrelia* species and STARI at the time of this writing.

- More *Borrelia* species and other pathogens that cause TBD are being discovered almost every year.

With such ambiguity and lack of easy and accurate detection, prophylaxis is the best way to protect yourself against the development of TBD. Starting herbal antibiotic prophylaxis immediately after a tick bite (or having it already in your system—see the following discussion of prophylaxis for high-risk populations) activates the immune system and initiates an antimicrobial response that will help destroy any pathogens that may be transmitted to you from the tick." (8)

This book goes into a lot of detail about how to make your own (prophylaxis) and is well worth the read.

The final repellant I will be telling you about has become pretty much the Gold standard and it will be covered in the next chapter on "Permethrin."

Chapter 6

Permethrin is the Best

In the world of tick and insect repellants, Permethrin is so special I had to give it a chapter all by its self. The following are a few reasons it is so unique and held in such high regard by outdoor workers, hunters, backpackers, campers, and all kinds of outdoor enthusiasts.

1. It not only repels ticks and insects, but it actually will kill them too.

2. It works as a contact repellant, meaning that ticks and insects don't notice it until they come in "contact" with it. Most all other repellants work by their smell, scent, or their aromas.

3. Just spray it on your clothes, shoes, and gear etc. (outdoors) or on a clothes line or flat on the ground. Next, just let dry 2-4 hours or best overnight.

4. It will dry odorless, so even hunters love it.

5. One of my favorite features is that when it is sprayed on clothes, it actually binds to the fabric and will stay there through many times laundering. It will actually remain effective for months and months depending on the mixture that you use.

6. It is such a cool product I call it "vitamin P" for your clothes because your clothes love it!

7. It is also non-flammable, so workers with FR (fire resistant) clothes like it too.

To get the most complete protection available, it is recommended to use Deet, Picardin, IR3535, or Oil of Lemon Eucalyptus on your skin along with permethrin on your clothes and gear. That combination will give you the best fighting chance against the pesky little mosquitos, ticks, chiggers, and other tiny bugs.

Permethrin application options:

- Spray it right on clothes and gear. It will not hurt any kind of fabric.

- You can pour some in a plastic bag and let it soak in on its own one garment at a time. This method is very effective but can be a little messy and is not used very much.

- You can buy pre-treated clothes that claim to last up to 50 washes or more.

- You can send in your clothes to Insect Shield to be treated to last for up to 50 washes or so. People have told me that in reality they may last about 2 years.

I personally like to spray my own clothes and then mark down the date. This method takes out the guess work and I know where I stand. I always want my permethrin to be at its highest level of protection because Lyme disease is nothing to play around with. Best storage methods for treated clothes are in a dark place away from sunlight in a black plastic bag. Also, do not dry clean treated clothes or they will lose their effectiveness.

PERMETHRIN FACT SHEET
DID YOU KNOW??

WHAT IS PERMETHRIN?

- It is a stable (synthetic) form of an insecticidal compound produced by the chrysanthemum flower.
- It is commonly used to treat lice (Nix 1% shampoo) and scabies infections (5% cream).
- It biodegrades quickly in contact with soil and water.
- It is odorless and will not stain clothing.

HOW WELL DOES IT WORK?

- It has been used as a clothing treatment to prevent bites from ticks, flies, and mosquitoes since the 1970s, and used by the military since the 1990s.
- It provides a quick tick knock-down effect – both repels and kills.
- A URI study found that people wearing permethrin-treated sneakers and socks were 73.6 times less likely to have a tick bite than those wearing untreated footwear.
- Each at-home treatment lasts for roughly 3-4 weeks (with washing!).
- Commercially-treated clothes can last up to 70 washes.

SHOULD I BE CONCERNED ABOUT USING THIS CHEMICAL?

- Permethrin is over 2,250 times more toxic to ticks than humans.
- Put directly on the skin, typically less than 1% of active ingredient is absorbed into the body; DEET can be absorbed at over 20 times that rate.
- Exposure risk of permethrin-treated clothing to toddlers is 27 times below the EPA's Level of Concern (LOC).
- A 140-pound person would have no adverse health effects if exposed to 32 grams of permethrin/day. There is less than 1 gram of permethrin in an entire bottle of clothing treatment.
- Permethrin is pregnancy category B (showing no evidence of harm to fertility or fetus).

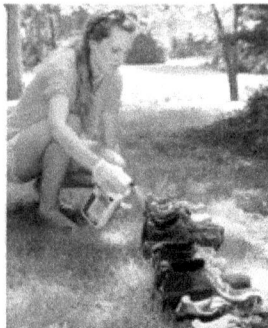

Caution: Permethrin won't hurt humans or dogs but it is harmful to bees, fish, and aquatic insects – do not spray clothing near flowers or water sources. Do not allow cats near permethrin-treated clothing until it has fully dried.

Treating your shoes with permethrin repellent is TickSmart and should be done every month throughout the spring and summer.

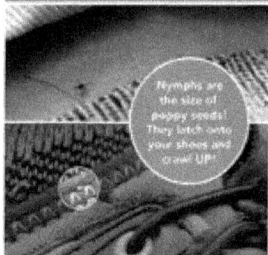

Nymphs are the size of poppy seeds! They latch onto your shoes and crawl UP!

Sources
United States Environmental Protection Agency. 2006. Permethrin Facts. http://www.epa.gov/oppsrrd1/REDs/factsheets/permethrin_fs.htm
Toynton K, Luukinen B, Buhl K, Stone D. 2009. Permethrin General Fact Sheet. National Pesticide Information Center, Oregon State University Extension Services. http://npic.orst.edu/factsheets/PermGen.html
Miller NJ, Rainone EE, Dyer MC, Gonzalez MC, Mather TN. 2011. Tick bite protection with permethrin-treated summer-weight clothing. J Med Entomol. 48(2):327-333 http://www.tickencounter.org/pub/tick_repellent_clothing.pdf

Tick Encounter Resource Center 2012

(1)

66

Tick Bite Prevention

The CDC recommends the following for preventing tick bites:

1. Know where to expect ticks. Ticks live in grassy, brushy, or wooded areas, or on animals. Spending time outside, walking your dog, camping, gardening, or hunting could bring you in close contact with ticks. Many people get ticks in their own yard or neighborhood. Soft ticks that spread tick-borne relapsing fever (TBRF) most often live in caves and rodent-infested rustic cabins.

2. Use Environmental Protection Agency (EPA)-registered insect repellents containing DEET, picaridin, IR3535, oil of lemon eucalyptus, para-menthane-diol, or 2- undecanone. Treat clothing and gear, such as boots, pants, socks and tents with products containing 0.5% permethrin.

3. Treat dogs and cats for ticks as recommended by a veterinarian.

4. Check for ticks daily, especially under the arms, in and around the ears, inside the belly button, behind the knees, between the legs, around the

waist, and on the hairline and scalp.

5. Shower soon after being outdoors. (2)

Permethrin comes in 3 different forms for application.

1. Aerosol sprays—good for 2-6 weeks and 2-6 washes note: protection periods vary with brand names.

2. Water based premixed pump sprays—good for 6 weeks and 6 washes.

3. Duration 10% Concentrate (the only concentrate made for clothes) to be mixed as needed and good for 3-24 weeks and 3-24 washes.

If you are considering the difference between the aerosol and the water based, I would suggest the water-based mixture. The reason is that most aerosols come out more airy vs the water based that comes out thicker. Therefore, more permethrin will be hitting the clothing, so more protection for you.

The most popular form used is probably the water based premixed pump spray because it is so simple to use. All you do is just shake the bottle and then spray it on your garments or gear. Let it dry and you are good to go.

As previously stated, it is always recommended to spray your clothes before putting them on and let them dry for 2-4 hours or best overnight. However, I do know of some outdoor workers who will spray down their pants (while wearing them) just before they walk into tick habitat. So it will work wet as well as dry, even though it will be a little damp and cumbersome. Keep in mind when used in this fashion, it is generally sprayed on more lightly, making it much harder to reach the whole garment because of the wrinkles. Because of this, it is often less effective. I get the question occasionally about this scenario, so I bring it up now because it's not mentioned on the bottle.

My favorite that I personally use is the Duration 10% concentrate where I mix it myself for whatever my needs are. It's so simple to use even I can handle the mixing process.

The product box comes with an 8oz bottle of 10% permethrin concentrate, a measuring cup, a 32 oz spray bottle, and mixing instructions. I normally mix my spray bottle with enough concentrate per the instructions so my clothes are protected for 12 weeks and 12 washes. This is double the protection period that any other product can offer. I like how it puts me in control of how long I want it to last. Basically, if I mix a little of the concentrate, it will last for 3 weeks and 3 washes. If I mix a lot, it will last for 24 weeks and 24 washes. Best part is this cuts my permethrin cost by about 50% because I do the mixing. See the following product picture from my website.

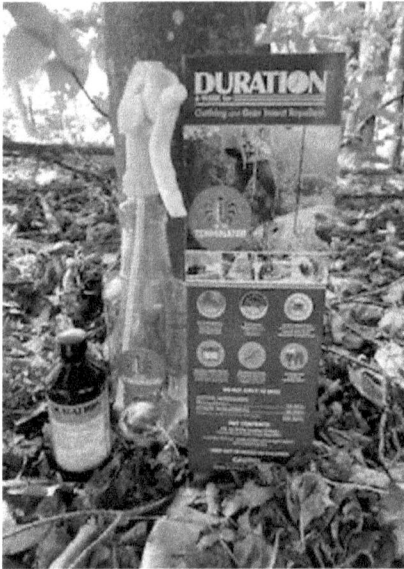

When spraying your clothes, always spray it on heavily so your clothes change color and look visibly damp. The heavier it is sprayed, the better chance it has to last for its intended protection period because then more permethrin is getting on your clothes.

Permethrin can be sprayed on all kinds of different things as long as there is some type of fabric for it to bind too. The most common things are clothes, socks, pants, shirts, dog beds, tents, bed netting, camping gear, etc. Some people have even told me they spray it on their truck door jambs (not sure how that works??) during turkey season. Others spray it on cloth truck seats, so there are many creative uses out there, too many to count.

Things to keep permethrin away from are cats, bees, and fish. I'm not a scientist, so don't ask me why on those, just take my word for it. You should also not spray it on your skin because it is becomes useless. If some does inadvertently get on your skin, the worst that can happen is a temporary slight reaction. Otherwise, just wash it off with soap and water.

Some of the permethrin views expressed here are my personal views and experiences from years of usage and feedback from many other people. Other similar views you will see are from Wikipedia, CDC, and Tick Encounter, which has all kinds of amazing info about ticks. In August of 2022, I had the honor of meeting with Dr Thomas Mathers, professor of Entomology at The University of Rhode Island and head of the Tick Encounter website. I enjoyed a fascinating hour and a half conversation with him and it was a highlight of my trip out east.

Always make sure to use permethrin that is formulated for clothes, EPA registered, then use as directed.

The below permethrin highlights from Wikipedia will give you some additional information on the origin of permethrin. Also listed are some other formulations that give it different uses besides the ever popular clothing tick and insect repellant feature.

"**Permethrin** is a medication and an insecticide. As a medication, it is used to treat scabies and lice. It is applied to the skin as a cream or lotion. As an insecticide, it can be sprayed onto clothing or mosquito nets to kill the insects that touch them.

Side effects include rash and irritation at the area of use. Use during pregnancy appears to be safe. It is approved for use on and around people over the age of two months. Permethrin is in the pyrethroid family of medications. It works by disrupting the function of the neurons of lice and scabies mites.

Permethrin was discovered in 1973. It is on the World Health Organization's List of Essential Medicines. In 2020, it was the 427th most commonly prescribed medication in the United States, with more than 100 thousand prescriptions.

Insecticide

- In agriculture, to protect crops (a drawback is that it is lethal to bees)

- In agriculture, to kill livestock parasites

- For industrial and domestic insect control

Insect repellent

- As a personal protective measure, permethrin is applied to clothing. It is a cloth impregnant, notably in mosquito nets and field wear. While permethrin may be marketed as an insect repellent, it does not prevent insects from landing. Instead, it works by incapacitating or killing insects before they can bite.

Pest control / effectiveness and persistence Permethrin kills ticks and mosquitoes on contact with treated clothing.

Permethrin is used in tropical areas to prevent mosquito-borne disease such as dengue fever and malaria. Mosquito nets used to cover beds may be treated with a solution of permethrin. This increases the effectiveness of the bed net by killing parasitic insects before they are able to find gaps or holes in the net. Personnel working in malaria-endemic areas may be instructed to treat their clothing with permethrin as well.

To better protect soldiers from the risk and annoyance of biting insects, the British and US armies are treating all new uniforms with permethrin." (3)

I hope this chapter has given you many ideas of how important, practical, easy to use, and necessary permethrin is in the battle with ticks for anyone who goes outside.

The next chapter will talk about what to do if bitten.

Chapter 7

What to do if You Get Bitten

I know you must be wondering, if I do everything right, I should not get bitten? In a perfect world, you may be right. However, in case you forgot, we do not live in a perfect world. So even if you treated all your outer clothes with permethrin, used repellant on your exposed skin, there is still a possibility that you could still end up with a bite. The chances are greatly reduced given your meticulous preparations, but it could happen. I like to try to cover every option so people will be ready for most anything, so read on.

When I give presentations, I always end with this subject because it is so important. I will normally tell my audience if you have not paid much attention to anything I have said up to this point, for your sake, please listen now. Note that all tick bites do not end up giving everyone some kind of tick-borne disease. However, in these next few pages, I hope to put the odds more in your favor, so read carefully, you will probably learn something.

First off, don't panic if you have just found one of those stinkin' little blood-sucking varmints trying to make a meal out of you. Actually, congratulations for even finding one from your tick check, because a lot of people never do. Does that sound familiar? This is another reminder. Don't forget to do tick checks!

Next, your first impulse will be to scream uncontrollably, then grab the tick with your fingers or have someone else grab it, yank it out, and immediately start smashing it with a 10 pound sledge hammer. I say instead: Hold on a second, try to take a deep breath and gather your thoughts because your next move is very important.

The way you take your tick off can make a big difference. Think of it this way "don't tick off a tick when removing them." In other words, be very gentle during the removal process. I know your first instinct will be to grab it with your fingers and pull it off, but please fight that urge if at all possible. Here is why: When you grab it, you will end up squeezing its whole body and that could inadvertently cause it to regurgitate (puke) some bad stuff into you. It's kind of like someone grabbing you around your belly just after you had a big meal. The best way to remove a tick is with a fine tip tweezers or a "tick key." I actually carry a tick key with me in my wallet because it is so small, flat, and convenient. The best tweezers I have seen are called "tick ease" I have one of those at home too. Both of those devices get the tick right by the head at skin-level without bothering their body or making them mad.

You also do not want to play with the tick, spin it around, put nail polish on it, Vaseline, or any of the other "old wives' tales." Most of those remedies do not work and only increase the irritation levels and give it the chance to puke that bad stuff into you.

Note the following excerpt by the CDC on tick removal and nice diagrams showing what I was just talking about.

How to remove a tick

1. Use a clean, fine-tipped tweezers to grasp the tick as close to the skin's surface as possible.

2. Pull upward with steady, even pressure. Don't twist or jerk the tick; this can cause the mouthparts to break off and remain in the skin. If this happens, remove the mouthparts with tweezers. If you cannot remove the mouth easily with tweezers, leave it alone and let the skin heal.

3. After removing the tick, thoroughly clean the bite area and your hands with rubbing alcohol or soap and water.

4. Never crush a tick with your fingers. Dispose of a live tick by:

   ○ Putting it in alcohol

   ○ Placing it in a sealed bag/container

   ○ Wrapping it tightly in tape

   ○ Flushing it down the toilet

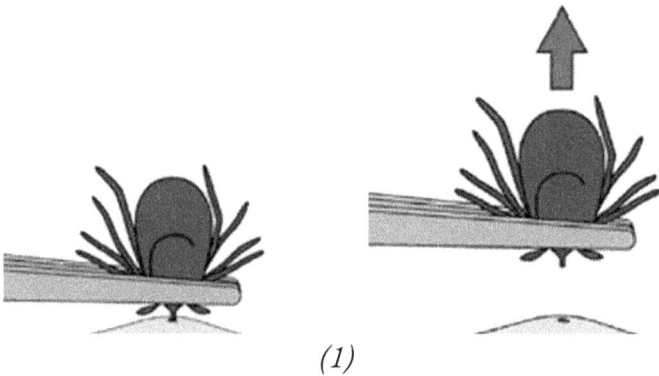

(1)

What you do with the tick is up to you. If you work for a company, be sure to know their tick protocol. It's not a bad idea to take a good clear picture of it and even save it for possible testing.

The next thing to watch for is the "bite area" and any of the following symptoms.

- Swelling around the bite.

- Bull's eye rash around the bite.

- Odd body rashes.

- Fever and or flu-like symptoms.

- Joint pain and swelling.

- Light sensitivity.

- Blurry vision.

- Partial vision loss.

- Hearing loss.

- Bell's palsy (where your face droops on one side or both).

- Headaches.

- Brain fog.

- Confusion or disorientation.

- Fatigue.

- Just plain feeling lousy for no apparent reason.

If you have any of these symptoms within days of your tick bite, **DO NOT** ignore them, but see a doctor soon. Note that different tick-borne diseases will cause different types of symptoms, which will then vary from person to person. Sorry, there is no "one symptom that fits all." So I don't care how tough you think you may be or if you just hate going to doctors, you better suck it up and see a doctor. If you don't, you could end up suffering for years or a lifetime with a bad tick-borne disease.

It is all about early detection and early treatment. Another issue to be aware of is if a doctor does not recognize these symptoms and tells you not to worry about it. If you get this type of diagnosis, by all means go to another doctor until you get some antibiotics to take care of the problem. Tick-borne diseases never get better on their own, they only get progressively worse with time.

As for tick-borne disease tests, the two most popular ones are the Elisa and the Western Blot. However, they are very often inaccurate with false negatives when the patient is actually positive and has a tick borne disease. The common problem is they are taken too early in the process when the disease is just getting started. Months down the road when the disease is well established, then they could show a more positive result, but then it's too late.

A lot of doctors who are familiar with tick bites and diseases will treat a patient early on by just the symptoms they show. This way, they will almost always stop it from progressing and their patient will avoid a nasty disease.

I want to say that I am not a doctor of any kind, but if you have read as much as I have, talked to as many people as I have, and listened to as many top professionals in this industry as I have, you would probably have the same opinions as I have.

Another thing to consider is if you are reading this and you are suffering with a tick-borne disease, it is best to go to a (LLMD) Lyme Literate Medical Doctor or some sort of "holistic" type of physician. Obviously, this type of doctor is much better equipped to help in this very tough battle, so please seek one out. Several top Lyme disease websites are ILADS, Global Lyme Alliance, and Lyme Disease.org.

Chapter 8

Conclusion

In conclusion, I will say my work is never done, ticks will never be wiped out, they are here to stay just like the mosquito. Like I have said, all we can do is protect ourselves when we are out there in tick habitat. We must also realize that their habitat is constantly expanding, so we need to be thinking and always be aware of them.

The following is a final, more in-depth list of occupations and activities that could bring you in contact with the enemy. When reading the list, I am sure you will say, "I never thought of that group" or "yes that group deserves to be there, that's for sure." So here we go!

All kinds of outdoor workers who come in contact with some form of tall grass, brush, or low-lying vegetation:

- Linemen

- Engineers

- Surveyors

- Utility workers

- Foresters

- Wildland fire fighters

- Loggers

- Tree cutters of all kinds

- Hauling firewood

- Oil field workers

- Landscaping

- Lawn maintenance

- Construction

- Railroad workers

- Pest control

- Ranchers

- Farmers

- Park rangers

- Trail builders

- Wildlife workers

- City and county park workers

There are all kinds of assorted outdoor activities you may not have thought of to be connected with ticks.

- Backpacking

- Camping

- Hiking

- Fishing streams

- Mountain bikers

- Jogging in the woods

- Horseback riding

- Gardening

- Yard work

- Golfing (regular or frisbee)

- Hunting of all kinds

- Hunting guides

- Outdoor outfitters

- Summer camp kids and counselors

- Outdoor education

As I close this book, I sincerely hope it has helped you to be more aware of ticks, their dangers, and how to handle them in a variety of ways. Also, do not let them stop you from enjoying God's beautiful creation we call earth.

For now, I leave you with my poem:

I hate them little suckers
I want to terminate them all
So I do it with permethrin
And love to watch them fall.

From head to toe I spray the stuff
My shoes, socks, clothes, and hats
Cause it works on more than ticks
Like skitters, chiggers, and even gnats.

So I ask you if you're listening

To keep away from Lyme

Get started with permethrin

And now's the perfect time.

Visit my website to get some great repellants, contact me for speaking, and more info on this crazy subject of ticks at www.thetickterminator.com

Thank you and be safe out there because ticks really do suck.

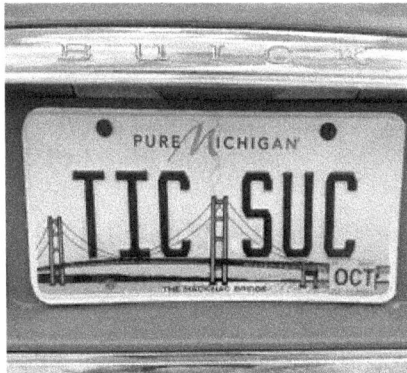

Source Notes

Chapter 2

1. Lorraine Johnson JD, MBA, Prevalence of Lyme Disease is a Big and Growing Problem—Let's look at the Numbers, CA, www.lymedisease.org 1/3/2019, website.

2. cdc.gov Lyme Disease Map, website.

3. Carolyn Crist, Insurance Data Shows Big Rise in Lyme Disease in US, New York: www.webmd.com 8/3/2022, website.

4. www.pinterest.com Frozen Tick: CG: credit: BM (with images) 1 Deer ticks, Ticks, Winter.

Chapter 3

1. www.cdc.gov Ticks Image Gallery, Tick Life Stages, Tick Life Series Illustration, website.

2. www.cdc.gov Ticks Image Gallery, Tick Life Cycles, Lifecycle of Ixodes pacificus, Illustration of the three year lifecyle, website.

3. www.cdc.gov Ticks Image Gallery, Tick Photos, American Dog Tick, Phil ID #170, website.

4. lymeticks.org Lymefacts, Preventative Measures, Diagram, Protect Yourself Against Lyme Disease, website.

5. www.cdc.gov Ticks Image Gallery, Tick check Illustrations, Tick check - Person English, website.

Chapter 4

1. Sean P. Ray, State to Study ticks in County, Meadville Tribune, Pennsylvania, The Herald, online newspaper, April 26, 2022.

2. Bronte Lord, One scientists radical idea to engineer mice and stop Lyme disease, CNN Business, 7/27/2018, online.

3. www.ivyoaks.com, website.

4. Molly Berg, UGA research links prescribed burning to reduced tick populations, UGA Today, April 30, 2015, online.

5. Shahla Farzan, Researchers say tick numbers related to local terrain, MO, St Louis Radio, 5/4/2018.

6. www.ticktubes.com, website.

7. www.cdc.gov Preventing ticks in the yard, Create a tick- free zone to reduce Blacklegged ticks in the yard, website.

8. www.cdc.gov, Preventing ticks in the yard, Create a tick-free zone through landscaping, website.

Chapter 5

1. Amazon, Lymeeze 3D Mesh Tick Repelling Leg Gaiters, online.

2. wikipedia, Deet, History.

3. wikipedia, Deet, Effects on Health.

4. wikipedia, Picardin, Icaridin.

5. wikipedia, IR3535, Ethyl butylacetylaminopro-pionate.

6. Insect Repellant IR3535 - EMD Group, About IR3535, www.emdgroup.com

7. Catherine Roberts, Ingredient Investigator: Oil of Lemon Eucalyptus in Bug sprays, Consumer Reports, 7/21/2022.

8. Alexis Chesney, Preventing Lyme and other Tick-Borne Diseases, Massachusetts: Store Publishing, 2020 print page 84.

Chapter 6

1. www.web.uri.edu/tickencounter Permethrin fact sheet.

2. www.cdc.gov Tick Bite Prevention, website.

3. Wikipedia, Permethrin.

Chapter 7

1. www.cdc.gov Tick Removal, How to remove a tick.

www.ingramcontent.com/pod-product-compliance
Lightning Source LLC
Chambersburg PA
CBHW060253030426
42335CB00014B/1670